P M S
&
Menopause
&
Hysterectomy

A Wholistic Approach

by Kurt W. Donsbach, D.C., N.D., Ph.D.

© 1993

Table of Contents

Table of Contents (cont.)

MENOPAUSE

THE MENOPAUSE

Menopause, often referred to as "change of life" or "climacteric," is that transition period from reproduction function to one of a more enlarged vista of activity. Most women, by this time, have raised their children, gained the experience that a lifetime of trial and error has taught, and are now ready to depart on new avenues of enjoyment without "that time of the month" to hinder activity.

Unfortunately, the woman who ceases to menstruate is often overwhelmed with physical and psychological phenomena which may make this time of life a miserable, tortuous experience. Since not all women go through this traumatic state, it obviously is not necessary and I will attempt to outline in this booklet the reasons for the problems and the means to solve them.

WHAT REALLY HAPPENS?

The average age at which the menopause occurs varies from 40 to 50 years of age, but the most common onset is from 45 to 48. There seems to be some relationship between the onset of puberty and the age at the time of menopause - girls who menstruate early often have late menopause, late menstruation leads to early menopause. There is also a correlation between women who have had multiple children and a late menopause. Celibate women also seem to cease menstruating comparatively early.

At the end of the reproductive period, the ovaries gradually become inactive. This process is the reverse of the changes that occurred at puberty, and a healthy woman on an adequate diet is as unaware of any disturbances as she was at adolescence. In some, the menstrual cycle ceases abruptly, in others, irregularity sets in for as long as two years or more. As mentioned before, some women sail through this change of glandular function without any symptoms, but all too often some rather distressing activities take place.

The most common complaint is that of hot flashes, involving chiefly the face, neck and often the upper part of the chest which becomes bright red and there is a sensation of heat and suffocation. These vaso-motor events can occur as many as 20 times a day and many times at night, depriving the lady of necessary rest. Sweats may follow the flashes or occur independently; at times so marked that the woman is drenched in perspiration, requiring a complete change of clothes. She is often especially embarrassed when in a gathering of people, she constantly wants to open the windows while the others feel cool.

Other symptoms often observes are dizziness, headache, difficult breathing or shortness of breath, and palpitations of the heart which make the patient apprehensive and very uncomfortable. Mental depression is one of the most serious of the symptoms, leading to shaky marriage relationships and friendships. Although every doctor sympathizes with the menopausal woman, it is difficult to really know how she feels.

MISCONCEPTION

The psychological changes which are present, such as depression, anxiety, agitation, apprehension, inability to concentrate, etc., are often brought about by a misconception that this signals the end of a woman's attractiveness to the opposite sex. Many wives are sure that soon they will age, with wrinkling of the skin, lack of sex drive, sagging, flabby flesh and a host of other totally erroneous conceptions. With proper attention to diet, skin care and muscular tone, milady can look forward to a number of sexually active years (often more than her male counterpart) with more physical energy than she may have had when she was menstruating and losing a certain percentage of blood each month.

Yes, the ovaries have stopped producing estrogen, and everyone knows that estrogen is one of the essential hormones that give woman her feminine characteristics. But nature is not so hardhearted that she would disregard woman after her childbearing years have ended. In typical attention to detail, nature has set up a backup system in the adrenal glands which begin producing a hormone similar to estrogen when the ovaries cease functioning. This hormone performs all the functions of estrogen except that of preparing for conception. And herein lies the basis for most of the difficulties some women have with menopause.

WHAT DOES ESTROGEN DO?

Estrogen is a broad term classifying several hormones secreted by the ovary which are responsible for the sexual growth and development which take place at and after puberty. They are essential for the development of secondary sex characteristics, such as body form and mammary glands; in the adult, they are essential to the normal functioning of the genital system. They are concerned with cyclic changes in the uterus, in particular those during the first half of the menstrual cycle.

In addition, estrogens bring about many other changes such as changes involving body form, condition of the skin and mucous membranes, structure of the skeleton, water balance and various other metabolic activities. Some of the most important functions of the estrogens involve their relationship to other glands in the body by antagonizing or holding in check certain functions of other glands of internal secretion. Thus when ovarian control is removed, some of the other hormones act in relative excess. Incidentally, this lack of ovarian function can come about normally during menopause or may be induced by surgery or irradiation.

THE PART THE ADRENALS PLAY

As I mentioned before, the adrenals are geared to take over the lack of estrogen by secreting a hormone which will perform all the functions of estrogen except produce the menstrual cycle. The only problem lies in an almost universal adrenal hypofunction. This state of affairs is best explained by the tremendous workload the adrenals have in our everyday life. They are the "fight or flight" mechanism that comes into play with each and every stimulus we have from our external environment. They also are very involved in our internal well being, such things as blood sugar control are related to the adrenal secretions.

Now for a moment think about all the conditions or situations which irritated you this day. Let me list a few common ones:

1. Children wouldn't get out of bed in time for school.
2. Children wouldn't eat what was good for them.
3. Children didn't dress as you would like them to.
4. Worrying how you can pay the bills this month.
5. Saw on TV or read of a murder, kidnap, rape or other crime which really upset you.
6. Husband drove your car yesterday and didn't fill the gas tank up, leaving you with just enough gas to get to the service station.
7. The appointment you had at 10:00 is 30 minutes away by car and it is now 9:45.
8. You just heard that in 8 years, the Social Security reserves will be completely wiped out. It will be another 17 years before you are eligible. What about all the money you put in?

I could literally go on and on, but the important point to be made is the constant stimulation which the adrenals are under. For each of the above hypothetical situations, the adrenals would have begun action to protect you

9

from harm (and you must remember that most of these are in the form of psychological stress). Creating a greater problem for the adrenals is a product of civilization.

A book was written called "Sugar - The Curse of Civilization" - later, author William Dufty wrote a mind boggling volume with the title "Sugar Blues." Either or both of these books should be required reading for all students of the art of feeling well. These authors tell the story of how refined sugar creates a very abnormal situation in the body which requires the adrenals to constantly be called upon to secrete a hormone which is necessary to convert a storage sugar called glycogen into glucose for fuel. See my booklet on "Hypoglycemia & Diabetes" for further information on this.

All this is only valuable to the menopausal woman to demonstrate the possibility of adrenal sluggishness at the time in her life when she desperately needs quick and active adrenal function. As the ovaries cease to function, the adrenals should begin secreting a hormone which will replace estrogen in the hormonal balance of the body. If the adrenals produce only little or perhaps none of this hormone, then we have the typical symptoms of menopause. The already tired adrenal becomes more irritable and the following are the symptoms of adrenal irritability.

1. *Dry mouth*
2. *Circulatory imbalance - chills and flushing*
3. *Temporary hypertension*

10

4. Internal nervousness and tremor

5. Abnormal perspiration

Do they sound familiar? Of course, they are the symptoms of the menopausal woman. The estrogen (or the adrenal hormone after menopause) normally acts to inhibit the sympathetic nervous system. Without this inhibiting action, the sympathetic nervous system allows all kinds of things to happen, such as blood, which is normally pooled internally, is suddenly rushed to the surface of the body, producing the typical hot flashes which are so annoying.

POTASSIUM AND VITAMIN E

It is interesting to note that potassium is a very important mineral for proper adrenal function and also for controlling our sodium balance. To be completely in balance, we should take in twice as much potassium as sodium in our daily diet. From all evidence that has been gathered, just exactly the opposite is true in the average diet - twice as much sodium as potassium. When sodium is overabundant, potassium is excreted out of the cell and lost through excretory mechanisms. Thus we may get enough of this important mineral in our food, but we have a sodium intake which is 4 times what it should be and potassium is lost. Drugs such as the steroids and diuretics also force the excretion of this mineral . Because it is so necessary for glandular function, the menopause may be just the time for you to look to your potassium intake.

Another factor which should be considered is Vitamin E. Although not reported in glowing headlines, medical literature is full of articles by reputable researchers who have found that Vitamin E is the most practical and effective treatment for menopausal symptoms, including hot flashes, high blood pressure, nervousness, heart palpitations, shortness of breath, insomnia, dizziness, fatigue and others. What is the possible mechanism which makes Vitamin E the key in these instances?

From a very scientific view, there may be no answer to that question. Some research indicates that all the symptoms listed above are alleviated in the menopausal woman who takes Vitamin E. The critics say there haven't been enough double blind studies. That is true, but the possibility of such occurring is very remote, since you couldn't patent it and make lots of money with the results. For now, we will have to take the anecdotal evidence and the scientific knowledge that tells us that Vitamin E enhances oxygen utilization in the body, protects us against free radical attack and stimulates immunity against cancer as reasons enough to use it.

STRESS PRODUCES SPECIAL NUTRITIONAL NEEDS

From a great variety of experimental stress circumstances produced in animals, we are capable to very specifically state what happens in the body when the additional stress of the menopause occurs in a woman. The nutritional needs will skyrocket, first in the particular needs of the pituitary gland, which is the "master" gland. Protein, Vitamin E, and the B complex vitamins are all necessary to maintain adequate supplies of pituitary hormone. Vitamin E, which is more concentrated in the pituitary gland that any other part of the body, is thought to be particularly essential; it prevents both pituitary and adrenal hormones from being destroyed by oxygen.

The adrenals are even more sensitive to dietary deprivation. A pantothenic acid deficiency causes the glands to shrivel and to become filled with blood and dead cells; cortisone and other hormones can no longer be produced and the many protective changes characteristic of the body's response to stress do not occur. Even a slight lack of pantothenic acid causes a marked decrease in the quantity of hormones released. The pituitary, adrenal and sex hormones are all made from cholesterol but, without pantothenic acid, cholesterol cannot be replaced in the glands after once being used up. If generous amounts (up to 3,000 mg.) of pantothenic acid are given and the deficiency has not been prolonged and severe, the adrenal hormones can be produced normally within 24 hours.

We cannot overlook or underestimate the necessity of monosaturated oils and butter in the diet. These are the sources of the sterol from which the hormones are made up of.

Although adrenal hormones can be produced without Vitamin C, the need for this nutrient is tremendously increased by the menopause and, if undersupplied, the

13

glands quickly hemorrhage and the output of hormones is markedly decreased. From experiments performed on guinea pigs, the need for Vitamin C may be elevated 75 times over normal during menopause. Translated into human equivalents, this means about 5,000 mg. daily of Vitamin C.

HERBS ARE ALSO VALUABLE

The natives of many lands do not have the modern laboratories to make drugs as we do and are forced to use nature as an assistant. Some of the herbs used through the ages for the menopause are:

Red Raspberry	*Sarsaparilla*
Cramp Bark	*Licorice*
Damiana	*Squaw Vine*
Black Cohosh	*Ginseng*

There appears to be specific action on the part of some of these <u>in assisting the adrenals to produce hormones</u> and others in acting as a general systemic tonic.

HOW ABOUT ESTROGEN THERAPY?

The advent of estrogen therapy was one of the greatest "symptom relief" therapies ever brought forth. Women on the brink of a nervous breakdown were miraculously brought back and became normal within a short time. <u>I must impress upon you, however, that very few miracles exist today - and the ones that do are not in the form of a drug.</u> Every miracle drug discovered is fraught with

14

danger, too often a danger which is not readily apparent. We now hear, almost daily, of the association of serious diseases with the use of estrogen therapy. Since estrogen has been used to induce cancer in rats, I would most sincerely, recommend that one improve their diet rather than resort to this method of alleviating symptoms. One doctor also stated that previously dormant cancer cells can be activated with the use of estrogen. My advise is to be very careful in using it.

LOOK FOR A PROTEIN SHORTAGE

A common cause of hormone shortage is insufficient protein consumption. An experiment was reported wherein good nutrition was substituted for artificially administered hormones. Of the 726 patients on hormone therapy who were considered, 81 were vegetarians, and 56 of these were willing to accept temporary addition of meats to their diet. In the 56, estrogen levels, as well as other hormone levels, rose in 65% when they began to eat meat. The vegetarians who refused meat were advised to cut down on cereals and cooked vegetables and concentrate on non-hydrogenated oils, raw nuts and sunflower seeds. When one to four ounces of nuts or seeds were consumed by them daily, there was a rapid rise to good hormone levels. Pumpkin, squash and sunflower seeds were rated most effective.

A PERFECTLY NATURAL PROCESS

Menopause must be considered as a perfectly natural process. Although a shifting of gears is required, no drastic symptoms need occur as the adrenals take over the production of a similar hormone to estrogen, which has been produced by the ovaries for over 30 years. This sequence of events should proceed calmly and comfortably in a healthy, well-nourished woman.

The body is marvelously fitted with a system of glands - pituitary, adrenal, thyroid, etc. - intended to manufacture hormones whenever they are needed, and in the proper amounts. This they can be expected to do, if they are healthy and properly nourished. When hormone secretions are inadequate, the usually reliable glandular structure is probably ailing. There are effective measures for strengthening the glands:

1. Researchers have shown glandular response to specific food supplements.

2. Since the cellular structure of the gland is controlled in its activity and ability to regenerate new cells, the DNA or "cellular blueprint" factor has been found to be of great assistance in rejuvenating an underactive gland. The DNA or "nucleoprotein", as it is sometimes known, is the intelligence within a cell which rebuilds an identical cell when a worn out cell is dying. It forms RNA which is then sent out to the blood stream for specific nutrients, such as amino acids, minerals, enzymes, etc., which are necessary to rebuild that specific cell.

In the late 1800's, Dr. Harrower first discovered that extracts of animal glandular material would help to restore human corresponding glands. Although DNA was not identified until 1960, Dr. Harrower and his work is still valid. Thus the use of pituitary, adrenal and other glandular extracts in assisting the body by the use of specific DNA factors to restore healthy function becomes a method of choice. These are available in tablet form in your local health food store.

SYNOPSIS

The following suggestions might be considered to avoid some of the "change of life" difficulties so many women experience:

1. Many individual vitamins and minerals are suggested as being helpful by many doctors, but I sincerely believe that a good high potency vitamin and mineral supplement will be more effective than any singlistic approach. I have outlined a formula which you might use as a guideline when shopping.

2. If anything is used as an additional supplement (to the multiple), you should consider Vitamin E because of the overwhelming evidence of its value. Many find that the amount in the multiple is adequate. If you do decide to use extra E, use the d-alpha tocopherol type preferably for a total of 1,600 to 2,400 total IU per day. (I have never found that this raises blood pressure as is so often cautioned.)

3. Herbs can be of amazing help in the menopause. The formula outlined previously has been used very

effectively.

4. A proper dietary program of food selection, with particular attention to proteins, is a must. The Creative Restoration Diet, which follows after the "Hysterectomy" section, is a common sense approach to this question.

5. The use of glandular extracts is also dramatic in the menopause. Again, I have outlined a complete formula of glandular extracts which support the entire endocrine system.

By following these suggestions, I feel that not only could menopausal symptoms be totally avoided when the time comes, but many individuals presently suffering can be alleviated of their distress.

STRESS PROTECTIVE NUTRIENTS

Vitamin A	25,000 IU
Vitamin D	400 IU
Vitamin E	400 IU
Vitamin C	2,000 mg
Vitamin B-1	50 mg
Vitamin B-2	50 mg
Vitamin B-6	100 mg
Vitamin B-12	500 mcg
Niacinamide	50 mg
Pantothenic Acid	1,500 mg
Folic Acid	400 mcg
Biotin	100 mcg
Choline Bitartrate	100 mg
Inositol	100 mg

STRESS PROTECTIVE NUTRIENTS (cont.)

PABA (Para Amino Benzoic Acid)	50 mg
Calcium	500 mg
Magnesium	350 mg
Phosphorus	100 mg
Potassium	400 mg
Iron	7.5 mg
Zinc	15 mg
Iodine	225 mcg
Copper	1 mg
Chromium	200 mcg
Manganese	20 mg
RNA	10 mg
Selenium	200 mcg
Valerian	100 mg
Adrenal Extract	100 mg

These are minimum quantities for a daily intake and some formulae may have added digestants, herbs and other food factors which enhance this product. Formulae such as these are available from your health food store or vitamin supplier, so read your label and get the best.

FEMALE
MULTI GLANDULAR

Adrenal	75 mg
Ovarian	75 mg
Thymus	75 mg
Brain	75 mg
Pituitary	75 mg
Heart	75 mg
Liver	75 mg

Pancreas	75 mg
Spleen	75 mg
PABA	75 mg
RNA	75 mg
Choline	75 mg
Pantothenic Acid	150 mg

Although still criticized by some, glandular extract therapy appears to be here to stay. I have used the above formula for many years in our hospitals and found it works remarkably well to balance the glandular system during menopause.

SOME COMMON QUESTIONS ASKED BY MENOPAUSAL WOMEN

Q. Will my sex life diminish after I reach menopause?

A. Although this does occur in some instances, the usual experience by women who take care of their nutritional needs, as outlined in this booklet, has been just the reverse. An increased freedom is often enjoyed because of lack of need to concern oneself with contraceptive devices and/or the possibility of pregnancy. There are also more days in the month that you may partake of sex comfortably.

Q. I seem to have a problem with a dry vaginal tract which intensified when I reached the menopause. This causes extreme discomfort in intercourse. What

can I do?

A. Although the estrogen hormone assisted in keeping the vaginal mucosa moist, there are several other nutritional factors that must be considered. Possibly the single most important is Vitamin A. It is the duty of this vitamin to protect and keep moist all the mucous membranes of the body. When it is deficient in the diet, or in supplemental form, an inadequate amount of mucus is formed which creates the possibility of inflammation, irritation, infection, etc. The United States Dept. of Agriculture study indicates that 50% of the American population are consuming less than the minimum daily amount recommended by the National Board of Sciences. The use of from 75,000 to 150,000 IU daily of Vitamin A will often relieve a dry vaginal tract all by itself. Another fat soluble nutrient, Vitamin E, is also often helpful. I recommend from 800 to 1,600 IU daily.

Q. It is true that after menopause, women begin to lose calcium from their bones and become osteoporotic (thin, weak bones)?

A. I do not believe that the advent of the menopause has anything to do with the osteoporosis which is often evident in older females. The loss of enough calcium to produce osteoporosis is something which takes much time and is often begun in the late teens or early twenties. It is a well known fact that the body will rob the bones of calcium in order to satisfy other more important needs. We also know that vigorous exercise and lifting or jarring-type work makes the bones grow stronger and denser. Women who exercise in any of the running, jumping, skipping sports very rarely have osteoporosis. When this disease is evident, it is the result of many years of robbing your calcium bank without adequate replacement from your nutritional paycheck. The use of calcium rich foods, a food supplement containing some Vitamin D, magnesium, phosphorus, plus the all important calcium can prevent this from occurring. Current medical treatment is the use of Vitamin D prescribed by your doctor but, I would like to point out that this vitamin is not a prescription item and can be purchased over the counter at any health food store or other store selling nutritional supplements.

You might also consider the sun - our most abundant and least costly source of Vitamin D. Use high calcium foods, a good all-around food supplement and try exercising in such a way that there is a certain amount of light jarring to the bony structure of the body. Skipping rope, volleyball, tennis, any type of dancing that is not just gliding or sliding on the floor, jogging, and rapid walking are all examples of easy to do exercising forms that will accomplish this. Such a program should guarantee that you will not suffer from the dowagers hump (due to collapsed bodies of the upper dorsal vertebrae) or fracture your hip from a rather insignificant bump or fall.

Q. Will my skin start to wrinkle now that I am not producing estrogen?

A. There is no reason for your skin to wrinkle any faster now than it has in the past. There are two primary nutritional factors which have to do with the presence or absence of wrinkles. Number one is protein. The skin is primarily a collagen protein substance which will break its continuity if you do not supply it with adequate protein with which to rebuild itself. This can be due to an inadequate amount of protein intake or due to a lack of protein assimilation. If it is the latter, a good digestive enzyme supplement is often the answer. I suggest you ask yourself if you have frequent indigestion, a growing dislike for protein foods (meat, fish, eggs, cheese, dairy products), or have constipation alternating with diarrhea. If your answer to any of these is yes, you may need digestive enzymes.

The second most important factor for good skin health is Vitamin A. Taken internally in adequate amounts, Vitamin A can have your skin literally glowing with health. It also protects your skin from many of the external chemicals and contaminants that would prematurely age it. I must say that the single most severe aging influence on the skin is excessive exposure to the sun. Ladies, wear a protective bonnet when you are out for protracted period of times, or apply adequate sun screening lotion.

HYSTERECTOMY

THE FEMALE REPRODUCTIVE ORGAN

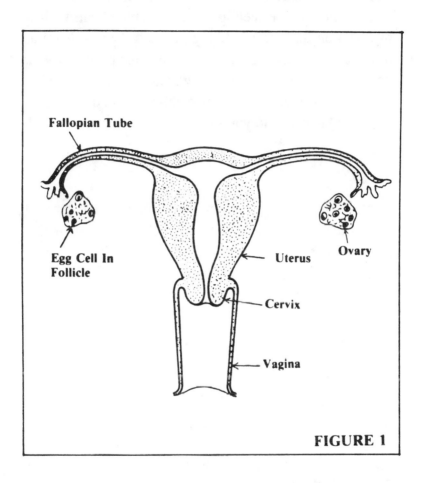

FIGURE 1

THE FEMALE REPRODUCTIVE ORGANS. The egg cells are shed from the ovary into the pelvic cavity. They find their way into the open ends of the Fallopian tubes and travel down to the uterus.

INTRODUCTION

So you've had a hysterectomy - like millions of other women. None of us feel good about losing organs and you might even be feeling uncomfortable about it. It is my opinion that the best thing you can do is to learn as much as you can regarding what has happened to your body. You are now a changed woman, but the world has not come to an end! There is much you can do. First of all, what happened to you?

WHAT IS A HYSTERECTOMY?

Very simply, the term hysterectomy refers to the surgical removal of the uterus or womb. There are different types, so lets review them:

1. Simple Hysterectomy - Only the uterus is removed.
2. Total Hysterectomy - The cervix is removed along with the uterus.
3. Pan Hysterectomy - Removal of uterus, cervix and tubes.
4. Pan-Total Hysterectomy - Removal of uterus, cervix, tubes and ovaries.

For your own information, you might wish to ask your doctor what kind of procedure was performed on you. It will help you to more thoroughly understand and apply the information which follows.

HOW ARE YOU DIFFERENT?

This is a very basic question that must be faced before proceeding with any sort of realistic life program. One obvious fact is that you are no longer capable of having a baby. That is a thing of the past. If you have had a simple hysterectomy and still have your ovaries, about the only kind of difference you will experience is that you will no longer have any menstrual periods. There will usually be no hormonal imbalances to contend with and there is neither physical nor hormonal interference with your sex life. Everything should be "normal" except for the lack of periods.

However, under certain circumstances, there are hormonal changes even when the ovaries are not removed. Hot flashes, emotional disturbances and other symptoms of menopause appear as if the ovaries were removed. After discussing this with surgeons, the most logical answer seems to be that certain blood supply routes to the ovaries are severed by the surgery so the ovaries are literally isolated from normal blood supply carrying nutrients to the cells and waste products away. This, of course, leads to malfunction. The nutritional management procedure, when this occurs, should be just the same as if the ovaries were removed.

Complications arise when the ovaries have been removed. If they have been removed, you are now in INSTANT MENOPAUSE. During normal life patterns, the ovaries came into importance when you began having periods. Remember how your thought patterns changed during those years? Your attitudes toward all sorts of things, including boys, suddenly took a different light.

The activity of the ovaries did this to you through their hormonal actions. You also developed physically, insofar as your body was concerned - hips, shoulders, thighs, tilt of the pelvis, breasts and a multitude of other physical and functional characteristics. You do not lose these functional characteristics. You do not lose these features now that the ovaries are gone, but the power that developed them is gone. In a sense, it is the use of these features that is altered, not that they are absent. For instance, you need not have a changed sex life because of your hysterectomy but, you will lack the cyclic hormonal influences you've had these many years.

Your ovaries also maintained a degree of influence over the metabolism of the body; the fullness of your skin, muscle tone, sharpness of thought, appetite for life and much more. You will notice a variation in some of these functions now. The variation is in the direction of aging. In one sense, it is the activity of the ovaries that tend to delay the aging process. The longer and stronger your ovaries produce in normal life, the younger you stay as the years keep rolling along. During the usual life pattern, decline of ovarian function comes on gradually. It is hardly perceptible until it is there. Your surgical menopause was not gradual, but instant. Suddenly, you no longer have the bodily influence of the ovarian hormones and yet the body is forced to carry on with an alternate plan of action, unprepared though it may be.

Another factor to remember is that this INSTANT MENOPAUSE has varying degrees of influence on you, depending where you are in the normal pattern of declining life. Are you in an age group where menopause is just around the corner? The younger you are, the more dramatic the change from normal hormonal activity to the alternate state.

PHYSIOLOGICAL CHANGES

To be more specific about the hormonal activities of the ovaries, one must mention that the ovaries normally produce two types of hormones: estrogens and progesterones. The normal functions of these hormones are:

1. to maintain estrus (menstrual cycle),
2. to prepare the uterus and body for pregnancy, and
3. to develop and maintain female characteristics: voice pattern, temperament, attitudes, body shape (hips, shoulders, thighs, etc.), breast development and other sexual individualitics.

Estrogen is more active during the first half of the monthly cycle, though present up until just before menstruation. It tends to rebuild the endometrial (inside) lining of the uterus. It also causes the follicle (egg sac) to ripen, ready for ovulation.

Progesterone starts its effect by causing ovulation or release of the ovum from the follicle and processing the endometrium to make it ready for implantation of the fertilized ovum. It works until just before menses. Menses occurs when both estrogens and progesterones drop to minimal levels and a fertilized egg has not attached itself to the wall of the uterus.

PSYCHOLOGICAL CHANGES

Obviously, these are physical changes which occur on a cyclical basis. There are also associated emotional or psychological changes which are normal for the various phases of the cycle. However, the emotional phases can become more than they should be when compounded by other stresses in a woman's life. Outside stresses make her much more susceptible to the inevitable cyclic stresses of her cycle.

Now that you no longer have ovaries, you are not a candidate for the cyclic stresses, but you are a victim of having no ovarian hormones, except for a small amount secreted by the adrenals which may be grossly insufficient, as compared to ovarian secretion. You now miss many of the systemic subtleties which have no apparent connection to ovarian function. Not only are there mood changes, concentration difficulties and other psychological reactions, but also problems with the system which controls your blood vessels; you have hot flashes.

To understand hot flashes, one must reassess the overall picture:

1. The ovaries have been surgically removed;

2. There has been a sudden or instant cessation of ovarian hormonal activity, INSTANT MENOPAUSE;

3. The thyroid and adrenal glands had no warning that such would happen, as would normally occur in a natural menopause;

4. Such a reaction is a severe stress, which shows itself in the strained reaction of the adrenal cortex;

5. Also, the thyroid is stressed so that it may, and probably will, work abnormally for a period of time;

6. These combined ovarian, adrenal and thyroid reactions cause an instability of the control mechanism governing your circulation, with resultant temporary flushing or hot flashes;

7. The same sort of picture can develop in the normal menopause, but one can question how "normal" such a reaction is, even though it is common.

Actually, "ideal" is normal and "ideal" does not include control mechanisms which don't work. Hot flashes, in the after-hysterectomy woman, are the result of absent ovaries with stressed thyroid and adrenal glands. It is a multi-glandular dysfunction.

Keep these concepts in mind when thinking about the INSTANT MENOPAUSE - several glands are involved and should be supported by multi-glandular therapy.

ALTERNATE MECHANISM

Normally, the body has a built-in alternative mechanism to be used in the transition from full activity to the alternative. First, there is a gradual decline in ovarian function, which lessens the shock of sudden cessation or INSTANT MENOPAUSE. Second, there are other sources of ovarian hormones in the body - the adrenal cortex glands. They have been producing hormones similar to those produced by the ovaries all these years without your knowing it.

The amount produced is only a small percentage of the total capability of your own ovaries when in their prime. But now, when the menopause is coming, this small percentage becomes a nice figure in reserve. It is a life saver which protects you from the effects of total hormone withdrawal. It is even helping you now since you have attained INSTANT MENOPAUSE. The degree of help will vary individually, since you are unique in yourself. It will also vary in effect, because of your own circumstances.

1. What was the situation of your life before surgery?
2. What was the surgical procedure like, and its effects on your body?
3. What were the anesthetic and post-anesthetic effects?
4. What were the post-operative medications, and how have you reacted subsequently to all these new variables (stresses) and to your changed life?

All of the above affect how your body will respond to its current status. One thing in common is that they are all stress factors. Stress is always a drain on the adrenal cortex glands since the adrenal glands are the headquarters for anti-stress activity within the body. Were your adrenal glands in good shape before all this happened, or were you on the verge of emotional problems or other physical problems? If so, then you can expect even more severe symptoms resulting from the INSTANT MENOPAUSE. Regardless, the current stress is one to contend with and deserves your total attention. It means a change in life style patterns, at least for a while.

Remember, no one else can make these decisions for you. It is your body and you are now in charge of what your body is to do and what it will receive. Unfortunately, you do not have the liberty of leisure during which you can do all the reading on the subject you may want to do. If you talk to the doctor, he will give you a more or less standard sort of answer about the usage of hormone substitution therapy and enough sedation to compensate for some of the bad times ahead. With this you have another immediate problem - are these synthetic hormones carcinogenic? "Will I get cancer if I take them?" This is a very real problem. "If the hormone withdrawal symptoms for the INSTANT MENOPAUSE are severe, do I take the risk of cancer or don't I? What are the relative factors to consider?"

These are questions and decisions you must make almost immediately, or perhaps should have made before the surgery.

NUTRITIONAL THERAPY

There are some alternate courses of action that deserve consideration. They work and should be investigated. Yet, there is little time for procrastination. You should have been presented these factors for consideration even before your surgery. The odds are a thousand to one that you were given even a hint that there were some sort of alternate choices. Ironically, it is possible that if such choices were made pre-surgically might have eliminated the need for surgery entirely.

VITAMIN E

The first consideration is - Vitamin E. This is a very controversial substance. (Incidentally, controversial drugs are not controversial or obsolete because of effectiveness versus non-effectiveness. They simply are caught up in a political battle.) There is no doubt in my mind that Vitamin E is effective in the menopause. Vitamin E is measured in international units, which is a measurement of activity rather than weight. My personal preference is d-alpha tocoherol, as this is the most active and effective.

Some recent work indicates that a dosage of upwards to 2,000 IU daily may be needed to allay menopausal symptoms. Vitamin E should always be used with

34

wisdom. Certainly, do discover what you can or cannot achieve on lesser dosages. Start with about 400 IU daily, then gradually increase the dosage as indicated. The one possible bad effect that demands alertness is an increase in blood pressure.

Literature talks about such a possible side effect but, in all the years I have used Vitamin E, I have not seen one case of Vitamin E induced hypertension. It may be one more of those unsubstantiated rumors started by vitamin antagonists to put fear in the mind of the potential user. Whatever the case, using 400 IU as a starting dosage and gradually increasing should be the standard procedure. I know one physician who uses from 1,000 to 2,000 IU of Vitamin E on all his menopausal patients with such good results that he has totally stopped using estrogens.

MINERALS

The next order of business is to balance the minerals in your body. This is called homeostasis - where all the various minerals are balanced between and among each other. It is a multi-faceted situation. Calcium is the one to consider first. A normal body needs about 1,000 mg daily. It is quite possible that your body, now in INSTANT MENOPAUSE, may need more than this suggested intake. Regarding the intake and absorption of calcium, there is apparently little difference in the source of the calcium since the acidity in the stomach breaks the bonds of the compounds so that the ionized form is passed into the duodenum. This ionized form is then chelated in the duodenum and absorbed into the system.

Chelation is the process of covering minerals with an amino acid cover to make them more readily assimilable. It would appear that 2,000 mg daily, as a supplement, would be more than adequate for the usual after-hysterectomy woman.

Phosphorus should be provided in a ratio of about 1 part phosphorus to 2 parts calcium, or 800 mg of phosphorus for 2,000 mg of calcium.

Finally, calcium metabolism cannot proceed properly without a sufficiency of hydrochloric acid (HCI), which is often depleted as we age. It is available in health food stores as Betaine Hydrochloride.

MAGNESIUM

Magnesium is very important to the body metabolism. It is involved in upwards to 70% of all enzyme systems in the body. It is, therefore, only logical to assist the body to metabolize normally by supplying an adequacy of magnesium.

Magnesium is available in many forms; magnesium carbonate, magnesium oxide, magnesium chloride, etc. Excess intake will cause a laxative effect (epsom salts is magnesium sulfate), but when properly combined with other minerals, this very rarely occurs. The need for magnesium is so urgent that certain medical researchers have administered magnesium intravenously with immediate and dramatic results.

Magnesium interacts with calcium specifically to relax and calm the nerves and muscles - in fact, is so effective that is has been called the "lullaby" mineral. The importance of this mineral cannot be over-emphasized, both because of its enzyme involvement and its relaxant effects.

Magnesium should be consumed at a ratio of approximately 1 part magnesium for 2 parts calcium. So if you are using 1,000 mg calcium on a daily basis, you should use at least 400 to 500 mg of magnesium.

POTASSIUM

This very important mineral is needed by the body in quantities 5 times as great as magnesium or 2.5 times as much as calcium. This should give you some idea of its importance to the function of the body. It works with sodium to form the sodium-potassium pump to introduce nutrients into the cells of the body and remove waste products. When this mechanism doesn't work well, cells lose their efficiency because of toxic wastes, and swelling or edema occurs. (See Fig. 1)

Another function of potassium relates to the all too often noticed phenomenon of intermittent tachycardia or rapid heart beat in the menopausal woman. Nerves pass their messages from one nerve cell to another by means of a chemical bridge called a neurotransmitter. Acetylcholine is one of the most prevalent of these neurotransmitters.

37

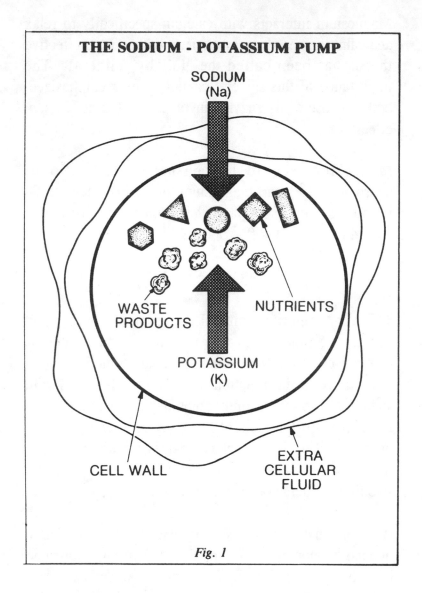

THE SODIUM - POTASSIUM PUMP

SODIUM
(Na)

WASTE
PRODUCTS

NUTRIENTS

POTASSIUM
(K)

CELL WALL

EXTRA
CELLULAR
FLUID

Fig. 1

The sodium acts to initiate the osmotic transfer of nutrients through the cell wall. Potassium, in repelling sodium forces waste products out of the cell. If potassium is deficient in the cell, sodium will enter and the cell is unable to properly dispose of its waste product.

38

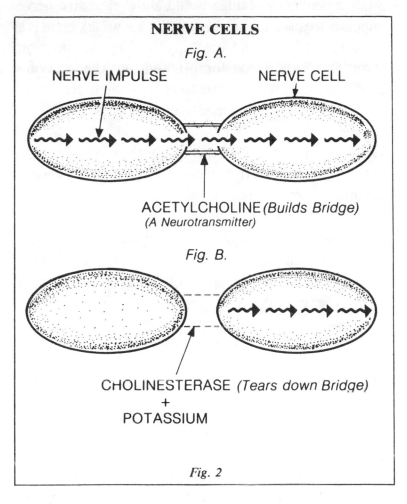

NERVE CELLS

Fig. A.

NERVE IMPULSE   NERVE CELL

ACETYLCHOLINE *(Builds Bridge)*
(A Neurotransmitter)

Fig. B.

CHOLINESTERASE *(Tears down Bridge)*
+
POTASSIUM

Fig. 2

A nerve impulse travels through a nerve cell, but must be transferred to the next nerve cell by a chemical bridge or neurotransmitter called acetylcholine. Once the message is passed the bridge is immediately disassembled by an enzyme called cholinesterase which can only do its job in the presence of potassium. These reactions take place in as little as one ten-thousandths of a second.

Since a continuous bridge would allow excessive nerve impulses to reach the source (usually a muscle), there is a constant "making and breaking" of the transmission circuit. This is accomplished by the enzyme cholinesterase, which must have potassium present in order to reduce acetylcholine to its component parts.

We can thus see, that in the absence of adequate potassium, the heart muscle may receive too many stimulating nerve impulses and beat too fast. (See Fig. 2) Fortunately, potassium is in plentiful supply in many foods, particularly vegetables, but if you are not in the habit of consuming a goodly amount of green and yellow vegetables, you could have a problem. I have found from experience that supplements of 1,200 to 1,500 mg of potassium on a daily basis will relieve most signs of this deficiency, particularly if vegetables are also consumed regularly.

TRACE MINERALS

Trace minerals are important factors in good health and are found in raw vegetables, fruits, nuts, and seeds. The trace minerals include iron, iodine, manganese, copper chromium, selenium, zinc, and probably several others which we know little about at this time. Only a few short years ago, we had no concept of the importance of chromium and selenium in our diet. Now we know that chromium is the center of the glucose tolerance factor and that selenium helps protect us against cancer. Studies on molybdenum, silicon, boron, and others are now offering evidence of their necessity in the human diet. Minerals important to man may be found in the multiple vitamin/mineral supplement suggested on pages 16 and 17. Auxiliary food sources, such as alfalfa and kelp, are often good sources of the more unusual ones.

NUTRIENTS FRIENDLY TO THE NERVES

As you are well aware, your nerves are involved in this whole picture. Nerves control every action of the body. You have been through a lot of experiences where your nerves have been abused to the maximum. It is only logical to support them by providing their "favorite nutrients" and to soothe them any way possible. They do not suffer from a deficiency of "Valium."

VITAMIN B COMPLEX

One of the friendly nerve nutrients is the Vitamin B Complex. This is a whole complex containing all of the B factors about which we know very little. We do know they are important nutrients. B Complex includes:

B-1 (Thiamin)	Inositol
B-2 (Riboflavin)	ParaAminoBenzoicAcid
B-3 (Niacin)	Pantothenic Acid
B-6 (Pyridoxine)	Biotin
Choline	Folic Acid
B-12 (Cyanocobalamin or Hydroxycobalamin)	

Synergistic micronutrients consist of minerals, enzymes, DNA, RNA, and many sub-molecular and sub-atomic factor about which we know very little. They are important because they provide the body with necessary ingredients so the vitamins can be metabolized entirely, without robbing the body of other needed nutritional stores. The B Complex family is usually found in cereals, nuts, and organ meats. Supplements containing B Complex are very common in the health food stores and come in a variety of potencies. My choice is still a broad spectrum multi-vitamin/mineral combination rather than purchasing everything separately.

LIPIDS

Lipids are the fats in our food supply - they may be saturated or unsaturated, depending on their source. These fats break down to cholesterol, triglycerides, phospholipids and are extensively utilized throughout the body. Many are not aware of the important part that cholesterol plays in normal nerve transmission, or in Vitamin D conversion from ultraviolet light. These fats also form the basis of hormones which control so many of the functions of the body. So, let us emphasize that the presence of fats or lipids in our diet is extremely important. Unfortunately, good lipids are not easy to come by in modern diets. Avocados, fresh nuts, eggs and raw cream are excellent sources. The essential fatty acids will be included in the above regimen. Highly processed, man-made lipids, particularly the hydrogenated oils such as margarine are particularly detrimental and should never be consumed.

42

PROTEIN

Proteins are the basic building blocks of the body structure. Our whole body has a protein framework. Proteins are also the basis for enzymes and some of the hormones. As such, it becomes obvious that protein in the diet is not to be considered lightly. Both quantity and quality are essential factors. Some amino acids, the constituents of proteins, are called essential because they cannot be manufactured within the body. Others are called non-essential but are manufactured by the body when all the essentials are present in adequate amounts. These "non-essential" amino acids are every bit as essential for good health as the "essential" amino acids, so don't overlook them. They all work together under the influence of DNA-RNA, hormones and enzymes to become the body framework or to be used for energy production.

In the INSTANT MENOPAUSAL woman, proteins are particularly important because of the immediate post-operative need for tissue repair and healing. They are also important because the immediate lack of hormones definitely hinders protein metabolism, and the body cannot keep up its repair and maintenance standards. The body tends to deteriorate more rapidly. Also, protein provides strong chelating agents (the amino acids) needed for proper mineral absorption. Finally, the potential lack of adequate hydrochloric acid in the stomach hastens body decline because of decreased protein digestion. In particular, protein will help you heal and maintain your adrenals and nervous system, as well as provide the basic amino acids needed to make hormones, in your case: corticosteroids, estrogens and progesterones, as produced by the adrenal cortex. If you no longer have ovaries, the adrenal cortex glands become "super important" for you.

DNA EXTRACTS OR NUCLEO-PROTEINS

Another area that can affect your recovery is the use of nucleo-protein extracts of glandular tissue, in this circumstance, the adrenal extract in particular.

The action of these substances is to normalize the tissues corresponding to the source: i.e., adrenal for adrenal, lung for lung, etc. Some may claim ineffectiveness since they are digested in the stomach when taken by mouth. True, they are digested, but the proper composite of amino acids becomes present in the blood after absorption so that the tissue itself can more easily glean sufficiency for rebuilding its own tissue. <u>It works and is non-toxic.</u> Excesses of nucleo-proteins in the diet are simply utilized as ordinary protein without any undue consequence. In your situation, your nerves and the entire glandular system, particularly the adrenals, certainly deserve all the friendly support available. For the glands, a multi-glandular approach is more logical: i.e., support them all. Please see formula outlined on page 18.

VITAMIN C

Vitamin C is used by every cell of the body, but particularly the adrenocortical cells. Vitamin C is ultimately concerned with collagen metabolism, which is the basic protein structure of the body. It also is involved with cementum, the substance holding the cells in capillaries together. In your case, it is particularly important because of its influence on adrenocortical hormones.

In extreme cases of avitaminosis C, there are splinter-type hemorrhages in the adrenal cortex glands, called Waterhouse-Fredrickson's Disease. Actually, the hemorrhages destroy the very cells that would utilize the Vitamin C to protect the body. These hemorrhages are also noted when cortisoneis is used as therapy, evidencing some of the abuse to the adrenal cortex by this medication. Mega C dosages are certainly indicated at any time the adrenocortical glands are stressed. In our society, our need is every day but, with you, who are suffering INSTANT MENOPAUSE, it is every day, plus, plus. This means you must mega-C supplement your body if you wish any semblance of normalcy. From 4 to 10 grams daily are suggested.

PANTOTHENIC ACID

Another vitamin specifically concerned with adrenocortical function is pantothenic acid. Symptoms of deficiency are usually mild and vague, like headache, malaise, nausea, occasional vomiting, accompanied by flatus, cramping in the abdomen and legs, loss of anti-body production and impaired motor coordination. There is a definite loss of stamina and integrity of the individual, which is really just a reflection of the failure of the adrenal glands. Pantothenic acid and niacin are both used synergistically with ACTH (adrenocorticotrophic hormone from the pituitary) in the substance used by the body to combat stress. Lack of pantothenic acid means a lack of anti-stress action by the adrenal glands. From 100 to 2,000 mg per day is an example of the wide range of pantothenic acid that can be used, depending on the circumstances.

VITAMIN A

Whenever resistance of defense is in question, one vitamin which comes to the forefront is Vitamin A. Due to the extra demands made upon the system to maintain itself, it may be wise to include Vitamin A in the supplement armamentarium, in dosages from 50,000 to 100,000 IU daily. This may sound huge to you, and you may be warned by some more conservative persons who really do not know from practical experience that such dosages are very valuable, yet innocuous and not dangerous. Symptoms like peeling skin and loss of hair can occur with much larger dosages. Even so, they are only temporary drawbacks and not permanent problems, as one finds with toxic drugs.

ADRENALS

As you noted throughout this whole discussion, the adrenals are repeatedly mentioned. They are important to you because they are the anti-stress headquarters for the body and you certainly are under stress. Secondly, they are now your only internal source of estrogens and progesterones. As such, they should be treated with TLC. Every nutritional suggestion mentioned herein has the adrenal gland in view, and you should too.

EXERCISE

Another factor which is not nutritionally oriented, but is wholistically important, is exercise. You should perform planned exercises on a daily basis. It does not have to be a marathon-type nor a back-breaking episode. It must be the simple utilization of your body on a daily basis. Keep active and you will stimulate your circulation, the all important lymph drainage, which relies only on exercise to pump the lymphatic fluid, and keep the muscles in trim. It is just plain common sense. Swimming, walking, jogging, running, and rope jumping are considered excellent types of exercise. The mini-trampolines are an effective, easy-to-use means of home exercise.

OXYGEN

The most recent exciting research I have completed began almost 10 years ago when I first contemplated the supplemental use of oxygen in a liquid form - namely hydrogen peroxide. Since that time, I have supervised over 150,000 infusions of hydrogen peroxide, talked to several hundred thousand who used the substance internally and am now engaged in serious work in the study of ozone which may be an even greater product than the peroxides as a source of oxygen.

So why should we make so much fuss about oxygen? The answer is really pretty simple - oxygen has two primary functions in the body:

1. **Creation of Energy** - This occurs when oxygen and glucose combine and adenosine triphosphate (ATP) is formed. Without energy, there is no life for life really is controlled by energy.

2. **Detoxification of Cells** - The oxidation reduction cycle in the human body is the great detoxifier. By combining oxygen with toxic waste products, less toxic and more easily eliminated products are produced.

Is there anyone who would not feel better if there was an increase in energy and there was less toxins in the body? Because of the universal effect of "just feeling better" that individuals who use oxygen containing products report, there has been a virtual explosion of interest in oxygen containing products.

These include the various hydrogen peroxide/magnesium peroxide products sold in health food stores, ozone drops plus some other not so valid products that have jumped on the bandwagon. (See my booklet on Oxygen, Peroxide and Ozone for complete information.)

SUMMARY

INSTANT MENOPAUSE need not be the living hell that many women go through. The following is a summary of the procedure suggested by the author as a common sense program of assisting the body to retain and maintain as near normal function as possible.

1. Follow the Creative Restoration Diet very closely as an every day eating pattern.

2. Incorporate exercise into every day of your life. If you value your good health, this is an absolute must, regardless of age.

3. Use a good multi-vitamin/mineral formulation and a multi-glandular, similar to the one listed, consistently.

PMS

NATURE GOES ON THE RAMPAGE

Jane, a 25 year old secretary to the president of a large auto parts firm, is a woman who describes herself as generally "talkative, optimistic and outgoing." She's pleased with her job, happy with her apartment and in love with her boyfriend, Dave. In fact, she says life looks great - until every month, about 10 days before her period is due, when she finds herself turning into another person. "My whole outlook on life changes," she admits. "I become moody and sullen, my skin breaks out, I gain about 6 pounds and sleeping becomes by favorite thing to do. As soon as my period starts, I am my old self - until the next month, when the same change happens all over again."

Jane suffers from premenstrual syndrome or PMS. She's caught up in a war being waged by her body's hormones and, like most women who get PMS, she has experienced the discomfort PMS causes. Sometimes its effects can be severe. For some women, intense depressions are a regular part of the monthly cycle, and suicides among women increase during premenstrual days. And, in a few rare cases, the irritability that is a common symptom of PMS, turns to violence. In fact, women in both the United States and the United Kingdom, on trial for violent crimes, have successfully cited the influence of PMS in their defenses. And in France, a woman who commits a crime just before her period can plead temporary insanity.

Though PMS is probably as old as the human race, it is only beginning to be researched and understood. Says Michelle Harrison, a Cambridge, MA gynecologist who specializes in the disorder. "Until very recently, it was ignored or trivialized as a silly female problem."

WHAT IS PMS?

In order to understand premenstrual syndrome one must understand the physiology of menstruation. It has been estimated that 95% of American women suffer from premenstrual symptoms at one time or another. Menstruation is a completely natural process and women experience it for many years of their lives. Yet, for a great number of ladies, it is a virtual nightmare. Menstrual distress is so predominant that it is known throughout the world as women's most common physical problem, with symptoms ranging from mild discomfort to severe mental anguish.

Many people, men in particular, have written it off as the "fate of womanhood," rejecting the need for treatment and women have resigned themselves to endure their suffering in silence rather than face the skeptical responses that are so common.

THE MENSTRUAL CYCLE

The reproductive period in the female lasts about thirty years. During this time, her reproductive organs go through a cycle which is interrupted only by bearing a child. The average female has about 70,000 egg cells in her ovaries at birth. These lie dormant until puberty. Then, driven by the anterior pituitary gland, the egg cells begin to ripen.

Egg Cell and Follicle - At monthly intervals, an egg cell pushes its way to the surface of each ovary. As it does this, it is encased in a covering of special cells. The developing egg in its cover is the Graffian Follicle.

The Endometrium Prepares - As the follicle with its egg cell ripens, the ovary secretes estrogen. The hormone, traveling in the blood to the uterus, causes the lining, or endometrium, to thicken and grow more blood vessels.

After about 10 days, the follicle splits open, sending the egg cell down into the Fallopian tube. The follicle cell, empty of the egg, then makes another hormone, progesterone. This stimulates the endometrium even more. It becomes very thick and spongy. Special nutrients are stored in the lining of the uterus together with many glands. The endometrium is thick and full of blood and food, ready to shelter and feed a tiny embryo. The egg, meanwhile, journeys down the Fallopian tube to the uterus.

The Fertilized Egg Settles - It has been fertilized by a spermatozoon enroute, the egg (now an embryo) quickly burrows into the endometrium. From the blood flowing so freely through the endometrium, the tiny embryo can take the oxygen and food it needs for survival. Eventually, a special organ, the placenta, grows from the tissues of mother and embryo. The placenta allows the developing child, or fetus, to feed on the mother.

The Unfertilized Egg Dies - What is the fate of the unfertilized egg? It dies inside the uterus. This happens to most egg cells. Only a few eggs are fertilized during the lifetime of one woman. After the egg has died, the ovary temporarily loses interest in the uterus.

The Uterus Sheds Its Lining - The hormones which were secreted in order to prepare the uterus for an embryo are no longer formed. The growth of the endometrium is dependent on these hormones. As their levels decrease in the blood stream, the lining of the uterus changes very dramatically. Almost the whole thickness peels off and is discharged. At this point, the monthly period or menstruation begins. The discharge consists of blood and tissue which was prepared for an embryo and which is no longer required.

The Cycle Repeats - The ovary produces ripe ova at approximately monthly intervals throughout the thirty years or so of a woman's reproductive life. Each time an egg cell leaves the ovary, the uterus prepares to receive an embryo. If the egg remains unfertilized, no embryo can develop and so the lining of the uterus is discarded. It is rebuilt as the next egg cell develops inside its follicle.

The menstrual cycle is interrupted only when an embryo implants itself in the endometrium so carefully prepared for it. Then the ovary produces no more egg cells until the embryo has completely developed and a child is born. After the birth of the child, the cycle begins again. It may be inhibited for some women by nursing, but this is by no means a dependable method of birth control.

Changes in the Breasts - The ovarian hormones, progesterone and estrogen, also affect the breasts, stimulating the glandular tissue. During each menstrual cycle, the breasts vary a little in size. They are usually largest just before the beginning of a period when there is the highest hormone levels in the blood.

Premenstrual Tension - The hormones have other actions and have a very delicate balance that must be maintained. Improper metabolism of the hormones or an imbalance of the two most predominant (estrogen and progesterone) probably cause all the symptoms we call premenstrual tension, or more properly premenstrual syndrome. Although research estimates of the prevalence of the premenstrual syndrome vary from 15% to 90%, it is safe to say that every woman has had premenstrual distress at one time or another in her life. It will occur in the fourteen day period before her menstrual flow begins and is relieved within one or two days after flow commences. We call it true premenstrual syndrome if it is constant and the score on the test which follows is at least a total of 15. Take the test and see just how severe your case might be.

TEST FOR PREMENSTRUAL SYNDROME

Instructions: Insert a number from 0 to 5 according to

the following criteria:

    0 Symptom does not exist

    1 Symptom is present but does not interfere with activities

    2 Symptom is present and interferes with activities but is not disabling

    3 Symptom is present and is disabling for one day per month

    5 Symptom is present and is disabling for two or more days per month

The following are common symptoms of the premenstrual syndrome. These will occur in the 14 day time frame just before your period starts and may continue for one or more days after it starts. If you have good months and bad months, try to average the symptoms.

_____ Nervous tension

_____ Mood swings

_____ Irritability

_____ Anxiety

_____ Headache

_____ Depression

_____ Insomnia

_____ Acne

_____ Weight gain

_____ Fatigue

_____ Confusion

_____ Increased appetite

_____ Breast tenderness

_____ Fainting

_____ Dizziness

_____ Craving for sweets

_____ Crying

_____ Edema (swelling of hands and/or feet)

_____ Forgetfulness
_____ Bloating
_____ Heart pounds
_____ Cramps
_____ Backache

TOTAL_____

IF YOUR SCORE WAS:

0 - 10	Very Mild
11 - 18	Mild
19 - 30	Moderate
31 and up	Severe

As we shall see, you can probably reduce your score with proper attention to both diet and nutritional supplement changes. Although a score of 10 is considered very mild, it does not mean that menstrual discomfort should be considered to be normal under any circumstance. With the advent of the recognition of the premenstrual syndrome as a reality, more and more research is indicating that the cycle should be relatively free from all discomfort other than the inconvenience of the actual flow.

Most of the symptoms that occur during the premenstrual time can be explained either on a very factual or a very educated theoretical basis. The following is the premise I used in formulating a nutritional supplement which appears to be very successful in preventing the symptoms from returning on a monthly basis. We should remember that it is not only the female who suffers with this problem - husbands, boyfriends, children, employers and employees all bear varying amounts of the burden. I recall specifically the case where one overjoyed husband came to me and said with enthusiasm, "You've just doubled my wife's pleasure. I love my wife very much, but she used to be with me only two weeks out of every month. The other two weeks, I was married to a stranger with an unpredictable temper and a lot of physical problems. Now she is even-tempered and lovable all month long."

HORMONES

During the normal menstrual cycle, two hormones have a great deal to do with the moods and behavior of the lady. Known as estrogen and progesterone, these hormones play definite roles necessary for the normal progression of changes involved in the preparation for pregnancy. The first two weeks after menstruation can be termed the "estrogen" phase and the next two weeks the "progesterone" phase. These time frames are, of necessity, approximations since it is the act of ovulation which really determines the length of the monthly cycle. If ovulation occurs less than 14 days after the menses, there will be a shorter cycle, or if ovulation occurs 16 days after menstruation, there is a likelihood that the woman involved will have a 32 day cycle.

Estrogen stimulates ovulation, so the level of circulating estrogen continues to rise immediately after menstruation until it peaks at ovulation. Then estrogen levels temporarily fall as progesterone levels rise. Estrogen acts as a stimulant to the central nervous system and is responsible, to some extent, for the feeling of energy some women report during the first two weeks.

Progesterone, on the other hand, is a central nervous system depressant and tends to have a calming effect. It should now become easier to understand that if the balance between these two hormones is lost, nervous symptoms can readily occur. Since depression is potentially more dangerous to life, after a temporary dip in concentration at ovulation, estrogen levels once again increase to balance out the progesterone.

Dr. Hans Selye, the author of the most authoritative research work on stress and its effect on the body, considers excess estrogens as stressors - substances that produce stress reactions in the body. If estrogen is not broken down in the liver properly, serious stress responses occur which result in some of the symptomatology of the premenstrual syndrome.

ESTROGEN USE

Estrogen (Estradiol) > Estrone > Estriol

Above occurs in the liver
Absolutely essential that adequate amounts of the following B-Complex are present:

A. Choline
B. Pyridoxine

If estrogen is not broken down in Estriol, Estrogen will migrate to target fat cells, primarily in the breasts and the uterus where the estrogen receptors are.

Excess estrogen produces:

A. Salt retention leading to edema or water retention
  1. Increase in weight
  2. Bloating sensation
  3. Pressure headaches from fluid accumulation in the brain

B. Increased levels of adrenal hormones which may lead to:
  1. Hypoglycemia, which produces
    a. Nervousness
    b. Irritability
    c. Weakness
    d. Faint of dizzy feeling
    e. Heart palpitations

All of this because of a lack of one or two essential nutrients! Maybe your understanding of the interrelationship of body function is becoming clearer after studying this illustration.

It can thus be seen that the B Complex Vitamins, particularly choline and Vitamin B-6, are very important if the liver is to regulate the levels of estrogen in the blood. Since it has an antagonistic effect to estrogen, progesterone is a natural safety valve in the body to counteract the stressful effect of estrogen. But even progesterone is not sufficient if the nutrition level is inadequate. The emphasis on over-processed, refined foods in our daily diet leads to a lack of the B Vitamins. The over-stressed individual is noted for making mountains out of molehills, they cannot accommodate to normal problems of daily living. This kind of "over-stress" can lead to even worse dietary habits.

THE "JUNK FOODER"

This over-stressed lady has a dramatic appetite increase from 10 days to 2 weeks before her period. She has a particular craving for sweets, often chocolate. The history of hypoglycemia would lead us to the conclusion that the mood swings from ecstatic to "bombed out" depression can occur from such binging. This revolves around the availability of glucose to the brain cells and muscle cells. The individual who is an over-consumer of sweets also replaces nutrient rich foods with these "foodless" concentrated carbohydrates that only offer glucose value and nothing else.

Thus, other very important nutrients that control certain emotions can be affected. Let's take a look at some of the very important protein derived amino acids and their effect on brain hormones.

Phenylalanine > is a precursor of > Norepinephrine
This brain chemical is responsible for a euphoric "feel good" sensation, for the drive necessary to complete work, and has been hailed as the best anti-depressant available. Obviously, inadequate amounts of

phenylalanine (derived from protein foods) would result in inadequate amounts of norepinephrine.

Tyrosine > is a precursor of > Dopamine

This chemical is responsible for mental alertness, appetite suppression, proper elimination of fluids from the body, and helps to eliminate salt. Tyrosine, like phenylalanine, is an important amino acid which requires adequate protein in the diet.

High levels of sugar in the diet cause another amino acid - tryptophan - to be forced into the brain cells where it acts as the precursor for the brain chemical serotonin. Like all other substances, serotonin has a beneficial effect but, when found in excess quantities, it stimulates the release of a hormone (ACTH), causes nervous tension, palpitation of the heart, and drowsiness with an inability to concentrate.

The very symptoms produced by the high sugar levels often stimulate the individual to eat even more sugar and the vicious circle is completed. If the individual is glucose intolerant or sensitive, they will produce excessive amounts of insulin, which further compounds the problem. To reduce this hyper-insulin response, certain nutrients such as zinc, magnesium, chromium, Vitamin B-6 and Vitamin C are of great benefit.

This chart gives some very interesting statistics as to the sugar consumption of women who suffered with premenstrual syndrome as compared to those who did not complain. The amount of refined carbohydrates was almost 200% greater and the equivalent amounts of refined sugar was almost 300% greater. Certainly such variations must have some influence on body chemistry.

DAILY INTAKE OF MACRONUTRIENTS BY NORMAL WOMEN AND PMS PATIENTS

Nutrient	Normal Women X ± SE	PMS Patients X ± SE
Calories % RDA	109.0 ± 9.2	139.0 ± 15
Carbohydrate % RDA	86.0 ± 6.0	107.0 ± 13
Carbohydrate % Refined	29.0 ± 4.0	47.0 ± 3.1
Refined Sugar (TSF Equivalents)	7.2 ± 1.3	20.0 ± 3.6
% Calories % RDA	41.0 ± 1.4	262.0 ± 29.0

DAILY INTAKE OF MINERALS BY NORMAL WOMEN AND PMS PATIENTS

Mineral	Normal Women (14) X ± SE	PMS Patients (39) X ± SE
Calcium	1390 ± 144	1400 ± 190
Magnesium	475 ± 69	367 ± 42
Sodium	2600 ± 300	4640 ± 600
Potassium	3770 ± 301	3700 ± 380
Iron (MGM)	34.0 ± 6.8	16.0 ± 1.8
Copper (MGM)	3.7 ± 0.6	2.4 ± 0.27
Manganese (MGM)	18.0 ± 5.0	4.1 ± 0.6
Zinc (MGM)	31.0 ± 4.1	15.0 ± 1.7
Chromium (μGM)	194.0 ± 38.0	165.0 ± 19.0
Selenium (μGM)	155.0 ± 19.0	158.0 ± 16.0

Figure 3

DAILY INTAKE OF B-VITAMINS
BY NORMAL WOMEN AND PMS PATIENTS
(Express in Mg/Day)

Vitamin	Normal Women (14) X ± SE	PMS Patients (39) X ± SE
Thiamine	76 ± 20	1.7 ± 0.25
Riboflavin	74 ± 19	1.6 ± 0.28
Niacin	144 ± 32	24.0 ± 2.4
Pantothenic Acid	173 ± 78	15.0 ± 3.0
Pyridoxine	104 ± 32	2.8 ± 0.4

From Goei G., Ralston, J. and Abraham G.E. J. *AppL Nut*: 34:4, 1982

FLUID RETENTION

Some who suffer with premenstrual syndrome complain of weight gain during the days preceding periods, with swelling of the face, hands and feet. The feeling of being a blimp with clothes, shoes and jewelry not fitting are hardly conductive to feeling fine. Others complain of increased size of both the abdomen and breasts. Most of the time, this is strictly due to an inability to release fluids from the body and can easily be controlled by some very simple dietary and nutritional measures. The scenario producing this water retention has to go back to the excess estrogen situation previously discussed. Excess estrogen releases stress hormones from the pituitary which inhibit water release and sodium excretion from the kidneys. Remember, we also said that excess sugar in the blood literally forced tryptophan into the brain which increased the serotonin levels which stimulated the production of the stress hormone ACTH.

Another chemical which is very necessary for life, insulin, can also affect the sodium level in the body. Excess insulin prevent the kidneys from excreting sodium. So the salt and water retention is really the result of two potent hormones, ACTH and insulin, which are excessively stimulated by the over-ingestion of refined carbohydrates, as well as excess estrogen.

SERIOUS DEPRESSION

One of the very serious and even life-threatening symptoms of premenstrual syndrome is depression. Some lapse into a depression so severe that they seriously consider suicide as a relief. The deep depression is often preceded by lethargy, confusion and non-responsiveness. The sufferer becomes very withdrawn and does not wish to speak even with close relatives, much less a trained health professional. In most of these cases, estrogen levels were found to be low or very low, and this may be compounded with the presence of the toxic mineral lead. Lead affects the central nervous system and one of its most common symptoms is chronic depression. Another finding in lead poisoning is the blocking of estrogen effect on target tissues.

If the estrogen levels are low, even in the absence of lead toxicity, then the depressive effects of progesterone will be unleashed full force on the female and there will be no balancing of chemistry. Although injections of estrogen will temporarily help this condition, nutritional balancing of the biochemistry is the long-term treatment of choice. If lead is a factor, the ingestion of adequate calcium can assist greatly, since lead accumulates in vacant calcium storehouses. Magnesium decreases the absorption of lead and also increases the excretion of this deadly mineral. Certain chelating amino acids, such as oysteine and Vitamin B-1, also have a great track record of hastening the excretion of lead.

HOW DOES MEDICINE TREAT PMS?

The "new" drug on the block is progesterone, an ovarian/adrenal hormone that balances the effect of estrogen. Since it is relatively ineffective given orally, many doctors prescribe vaginal suppositories, from one to three per day. Let's look at some of the effects of this drug.

A. It lowers blood sugar because it is an antagonist to adrenaline, which helps normalize blood glucose levels. Because of this, the menstruating female begins to crave sugar laden foods to bring up her glucose level. This leads to or exacerbates hypoglycemia.

B. If the oral, synthetic progesterone is used (called progestogen), it often causes water retention.

C. The use of progesterone in any form may inhibit natural progesterone production which will cause even more problems.

In addition, I would like to quote from *Medical Month*, an article entitled "Dangerous Fad Therapy for Premenstrual Syndrome." Quote: "Many gynecologists fear women taking huge doses of progesterone for extended periods, are risking cardiovascular problems, diabetes, and possibly even ovarian or uterine cancer. In short, we may be seeing the beginnings of yet another women's health disaster - a variation on the themes of diethylstilbestrol and high-dose oral contraceptives." Unquote.

The rational of progesterone therapy is based upon the fact that the premenstrual syndrome is really only experienced during the approximately two weeks before menstruation, and since that is the "progesterone" phase, their symptoms must be due to a lack of this hormone. The facts presented prior to this will show the reader how shallow that reasoning is.

There are many other factors involved other than inadequate progesterone. To further quote the previously mentioned article by Reni L. Witt in the February, 1984 issue, "Only natural progesterone, not the synthetic progestrogens in oral contraceptives, is considered effective. Explains, ob-gyn Steven Greenberg, assistant professor at Temple University Medical School in Philadelphia and founder of Focus on PMS, a suburban clinic, "Progestrogens take up the progesterone binding sites, blocking self production (of progesterone) and in effect intensifying the hormone imbalance. The synthetics also have estrogenic and androgenic effects that can worsen symptoms."

Other critics speak out loudly against progesterone therapy, pointing out that breakthrough bleeding is common while suppositories are is use, sometimes even on a constant basis. Some warn against the possible "withdrawal" which might occur if progesterone is abruptly stopped. Reports of migraine headaches, mood swings and a feeling of agitation after the use of the last suppository in the cycle certainly are cause for serious consideration.

Symptoms such as vaginal irritation, vaginal swelling, itching, uterine cramping, insomnia, decreased libido, as well as the very symptoms progesterone is intended to correct: breast tenderness, hot flushes, mood swings, fatigue, increased appetite and craving for salty foods are all a part of the side effects of the use of this drug.

Premenstrual Symptoms

A group of 150 women (100 college students and 50 registered nurses) were asked to fill out a questionnaire regarding menstrual symptoms. Here are the results.

Pain Before Menstruation					47%
During Menstruation					66%
Loss of Work (at least one day)					15%
Irritability					69%
Depression					63%
Insomnia					5%
Acne					70%
Face	55%	Chest	8.6%	Elsewhere	6.4%
Increase in Vaginal Discharge					49%
Headaches					32%
Swelling					
Abdominal	52%	Breasts	40%	Hands	3%
Feet	3%	Face	3%		
No Symptoms					3%

Source: A critical analysis of the Premenstrual Syndrome, Sutherland - Stewart Lancet 6-5-65 1180-1183

The tremendous impact of this response is that 97% of the menstruating female population has significant symptoms. Menstruation is and should be a normal function, basically asymptomatic. The reverse is actually true - almost everyone has such a change in physiology that medical symptoms are produced.

APPROACHING PMS NUTRITIONALLY

The treatment of PMS from a strictly nutritional point of view may be scoffed at by some and criticized by others. But let's review the facts:

1. According to the best research, certain symptoms of PMS are probably due to an imbalance in the two basic hormones - estrogen and progesterone. Some of the symptoms can be directly traced to an increase of blood

72

levels of estrogen. Under normal circumstances, the liver will degrade estrogen to estriol which does not produce such symptoms; in fact, it will prevent them. In the absence of adequate B Complex vitamins, the liver cannot do its job in breaking down estrogen.

2. Other symptoms of PMS are directly related to an increased consumption of refind carbohydrates. A study of the refined sugar intake of sufferers vs. non-sufferers of PMS was quite conclusive in relating high intake of sugar to PMS.

3. Some symptoms of PMS are probably concurrently related to estrogen dominance and poor nutrition. Hormone induced sodium retention can be aggravated by a sodium rich--potassium poor diet.

4. Without a doubt, there are some PMS victims who have a low progesterone output and may temporarily require medical assistance. But like all hormone levels in the body, progesterone is nutritionally dependent. If the raw materials are present for the body to manufacture it, and the gland which manufactures it (basically the ovary) is healthy, there should be an adequate supply for normal use.

So let's look at a nutritional approach.

A. Increase the complex carbohydrates in your diet.
Man was accustomed to a high complex carbohydrate intake for many thousands of years. Then one day, he found out how to concentrate the sweetness he found so

satisfying and we have been paying the price ever since. By concentrating on the complex carbohydrates (basically the vegetables, cereals and fruits), you will find that you desire the refined sugars less. In our two hospitals and one resort, we suggest that all our patients consume at least 4 cups of vegetables each day, preferably with at least two cupfuls raw.

B. Limit your intake of coffee, tea, chocolate, smoking.

These substances either contain or cause the body to produce deleterious substances that are associated with some of the symptoms associated with PMS. One researcher had some rather good results doing nothing more than eliminating these four things from the patient's lifestyle.

C. Consume adequate quality proteins.

A deficiency of certain amino acids can aggravate or even produce mood changes that are often seen in PMS. Quality protein does not mean to eat red meat, although red meat is a quality protein. You can get quality protein from a balanced vegetarian, lacto-vegetarian, lacto-ovo-vegetarian, or a fishy-lacto-ovo-vegetarian diet. It is known that the meats (including all fowl), fish, eggs and dairy products provide more high quality protein on a gram for gram basis than other foods. If you are consuming your four cupfuls of vegetable each day, it is unlikely that you will over-eat on your proteins.

D. Do use a food supplement that will encompass all the nutritional deficiencies which are known to be beneficial for PMS.

Nutritional supplementation is an exciting field today. Many physicians are finding that concentrated food supplements are providing them with more results than the drugs that are the foundation of medical education. The resistance that is shown is just an affirmation of the old adage, "It's easy to criticize that which you know little about." PMS responds beautifully to a nutritional regimen.

E. Do exercise on a regular basis.

Vigorous exercise is not necessary to get the benefits that are yours, free for the asking. A fast paced one half hour walk on a daily basis will provide you with wonderful physical changes that amaze most who have lead a sedentary life up to this point. You will find that there is certain addiction to this regime, if you miss, your body will gently chide you to "get with it." You can expect both physical and emotional relaxation, improved circulation, improvement in sleep patterns and, of course, improved muscle tone.

SUGGESTED SUPPLEMENT
FORMULA FOR PMS

Vitamin A	15,000 IU
Beta Carotene	15,000 IU
Vitamin D	800 IU
Vitamin E	400 IU
Vitamin C	1,000 mg
Vitamin B-1	25 mg
Vitamin B-2	25 mg
Niacinamide	25 mg
Inositol	25 mg
PABA	25 mg
B-6	200 mg
Pantothenic Acid	200 mg
B-12	500 mcg
Folic Acid	400 mcg
Biotin	25 mcg
Choline	600 mg
Calcium	800 mg
Magnesium	800 mg
Iron	18 mg
Iodine	225 mcg
Copper	400 meg
Zinc	16 mg
Chromium	200 mcg
Selenium	200 mcg
Potassium	400 mg
L-Phenylalanine	200 mg
GLA	200 mg

This supplement should be used on a daily basis as your complete nutritional vitamin and mineral support. The high **Vitamin A** content tends to normalize the production of estrogen and progesterone by its effect on the pituitary which, in reality, controls all hormone production in the body. Of all the B Complex vitamins,

B-6 is probably most commonly associated with PMS since it helps to control so many metabolic reactions in the body, not the least of which is water elimination.

Choline is a mighty liver helper and without this often overlooked nutrient, the liver cannot properly metabolize estrogen, leaving high blood levels, which result in the symptom pattern we call PMS.

Magnesium is called the great relaxer and Dr. G.E. Abraham of UCLA, found that blood levels of women with PMS were significantly lower in magnesium than women who did not have premenstrual tension.

Phenylalanine is considered by some researchers to be one of the finest anti-depressants available. Nutritional supplementation works best when all nutrients are present. It appears that the sum of the whole is greater than the sum of its parts. This does not preclude adjustment of certain nutrients, as in the PMS formulation, which are particularly indicated for a specific reason.

By combining all the elements into one formula, you save yourself the job of trying to find seven or eight different bottles which approximate what is desired.

CONCLUSION

The female has been, and probably always will be, the stronger of the species. To allow a totally preventable and/or treatable condition to influence your life in such a way that you are partially functional on a regular basis doesn't make sense. Don't let PMS interfere with your family or your work relationship. If you have it, accept the fact and do something about it.

SOME DOCUMENTATION

Improved PMS symptomatology reported in 84% of patients taking Vitamin B-6 under controlled conditions. (Abraham and Hargrove 1NF-3:155, 1980)

Improved premenstrual breast symptomatology in 85% of patients taking Vitamin E under controlled conditions. (London et al. - Breast 4:10, 1978)

Improvement of acne score by 85% in patients taking Vitamin A and zinc under controlled conditions. (Michaelson et al. Arch. Derm 113:31, 1977)

EXERCISE

Avoid violent, strenuous exercise. It decreases liver functions. Best and most practical exercise is FAST WALKING (4-5 miles/hour) outdoors for 30 minutes once or twice a day.

PMS SYMPTOMATOLOGY

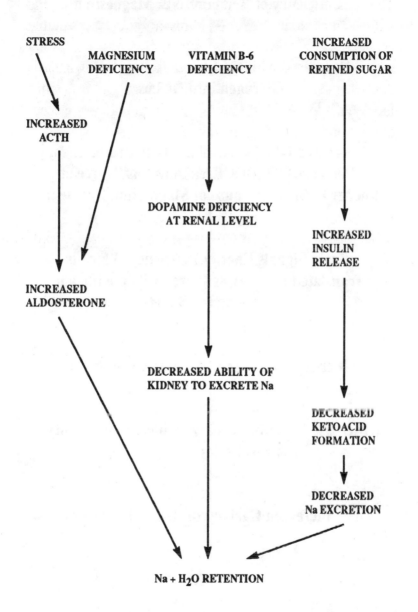

GRAPHIC ILLUSTRATION OF PMS

Deficiency of B Vitamins & Magnesium

↓

Decreased Ability of Liver to Break Down
Glycogen into Glucose

↓

Decreased Glucose Availability to Brain. Also,
Decreased Glucose Breakdown as Source of
Energy to Brain Because of Magnesium Deficiency

↓

Brain Signals Energy Deficiency Which is
Translated by Body as Increased Appetite and
Craving for Sweets

↓

Increased Consumption of Refined Sugar

↓

Increased Insulin Levels and Increased Affinity
of Insulin for Receptors

↓

Increased Carbohydrate Intolerance

↓

PMS SYMPTOMS

THE CREATIVE RESTORATION DIET

This message is for you! It is a health program designed for modern living, with a great deal of study and practical clinical experience resulting in this concise and precision-engineered schedule. Any program can only be as effective as its application. Anything worth doing is worth doing well, so why not make a real challenge to put it to work for a mere 30 days of your life and, in return, have a chance at increased health, the greatest wealth of all?

Incompatible With This Program

Certain habits are incompatible with your search for health. You cannot build with one hand while tearing down with the other and expect to fashion a monument. The following are incompatible with good health:

Consumption of alcohol Except in extreme moderation, the consumption of alcohol destroys brain cells and is very damaging to the liver.

Smoking So much evidence has been presented in the public press that we need not elaborate but, specifically, it is cancer causing, increases risk of heart disease and destroys Vitamin C, which leads to many other problems.

Over-consumption of coffee or tea Both of these contain habit-forming drugs and are deleterious to the central nervous system. You may substitute herb teas or cereal beverages available at health food stores.

UNDERSTANDING THE CREATIVE RESTORATION DIET

This is a recommended method of eating foods to induce you to "automatically" improve your diet. **It Must Be Understood**, not just blindly followed. You must learn to lead your own way. Unlike the dull, restricted menu-type diet which requires discipline to enforce, this educational approach can be interesting. It encourages a greater, rather than lesser variety of foods, thus both taste and appetite are more likely to be satisfied. There is also a great satisfaction in being able to select foods by reason of good judgement and common sense, rather than by the usual hit or miss method.

Therefore, please read the following information carefully. If you understand why you are asked to follow certain Rules and Guidelines, it will be much easier to gain your cooperation. It merely takes plain, common sense and a wisp of will power. Your conscience should become your guide. Since this diet consists primarily of vegetables, meat, cheese, fish, poultry and fruit, it is high in minerals, especially potassium, an essential mineral of prime importance in the body chemistry. Because it is high in fiber foods, which are both cleansing and speed up the tract time, it encourages a favorable intestinal environment. It is intended to eliminate a high portion of so-called "empty calorie" foods, so it should have an excellent *weight normalization* influence.

Naturally, all of the foods which one should not eat cannot be mentioned. Only the major classifications are mentioned in this regard, listing a few categories only. The guidelines for food combinations are few and easy to follow. Emphasis is placed upon the positive "what to eat" nature of dieting. It is a diet you can believe in because it is deemed to be right, founded in truth, rather than fancy or statistics. Basic rules to follow are listed at end of text. These should be learned and practiced until they become matters of habit.

GENERAL PRINCIPLES

Regarding white flour and white sugar products - not only are white flour and sugar products devoid of their natural occurring vitamins and minerals, but the less desirable calories are concentrated until they become little more than pure starch and carbohydrate. Why is this abuse of Nature's stores brought about?

In the case of the white flour, shelf-life is the main reason. All commercial white flour is processed so that it can be stored for long periods of time. To make this possible, most of the "life" is removed from the whole wheat berries. Since the oil is removed, it cannot turn rancid. Everything subject to oxidation has been removed. If it were not so, spoilage would be very rapid, often within a period of a few days.

White sugar is refined for another reason. In its liquid form as cane juice, it would ferment rapidly and would require refrigeration from cane field to user. Obviously, this would not serve commercial purposes. Granulated sugar did! But the attendant loss of vitamins and minerals, plus the intensive concentration of purified carbohydrate, made a mixture too rich to handle by your body, much like the carburetor on your car when too much gas is mixed with the air.

An important feature of the Creative Restoration Diet is to *eat maximum quantities of live foods and eliminate purified foods.* White flour products are dead foods (no enzymes and most or all of the vitamins and minerals removed) and are purified substances which the body finds difficult to adapt to normal metabolism.

It is comparatively simple to eliminate much white sugar from the diet simply by not eating candy, pastries and so forth made of white sugar. However, many find it difficult to eliminate all white flour products such as bread, bakery rolls, paste foods (white flour macaroni, spaghetti and the like). The elimination of most white flour products is essential, however, if the fullest benefits are to be obtained from the Creative Restoration Diet.

Regarding the Use of Uncooked Foods - Let's look at your diet from the aspect of how much of it consists of uncooked or raw foods. Many people go days on end with no more raw food than a smattering of lettuce or an occasional glass of fruit juice. The remainder of their diet is completely cooked! *The eating of fresh, raw foods daily should never be left to chance.* Two outstanding all-season foods are recommended as always being available: tomatoes and tomato juice and raw cabbage.

Although raw tomatoes are usually best, canned tomatoes, without preservatives added, are on the list of acceptable foods. Tomatoes are one of the few vegetables which lend themselves well to the canning process. In fact, because tomatoes are canned at the height of their natural perfection, the food value can be higher than the hothouse variety sold in off-seasons. The same applies to tomato juice with both offering rich sources of potassium and Vitamins A, B and C.

Salads made with raw cabbage instead of lettuce can be one of the greatest taste surprises you have ever had. **Cabbage in raw form is one of our richest sources of essential vitamins and minerals. It stores as well, if not better, than any other raw food, keeping its nutrients beneath its protective wrapper in the leaves.** *It is indispensable to the success of this diet that a high quality raw food be included in the diet daily.* Tomato and cabbage have been suggested, if at all possible, I use one cupful of raw cabbage with a little raw potato or jicima or water chestnut mixed in every day. Raw carrots, cauliflower, sprouts, celery, etc. are almost always available and can be used to excellent advantage.

Regarding Use of Meat Products Meats, such as veal, beef, lamb and chicken are good sources of protein. However, even though the protein intake is adequate insofar as quality is concerned, quality is an even more important point to consider. Incomplete proteins leave out pieces of the "building block" mechanism, and like a jigsaw puzzle with pieces missing, the whole picture suffers. This can be a good reason to supplement the diet with a multiple source protein product to assure an adequate amino acid supply and balance.

Also, in regard to protein ingestion, its breakdown into amino acids is essential to its utilization. This is called the process of digestion. If digestion fails to liquefy the meat (protein), spoilage can occur in the intestinal tract - a process called putrefaction. Effects of putrefaction in the gastrointestinal tract are bad breath, foul-odored stool and general decrease in energy. This is a good reason to supplement the diet with an appropriate digestive enzyme product, both facilitating breakdown of the protein and preventing putrefaction.

Contrary to some opinions, the grinding of meat into small particles, e.g., hamburger, does not increase its digestibility. On the other hand, grinding of meat can have deleterious effects. Ground meat spoils rapidly at room temperature, whole meat does not, in fact, aging of whole meat can make it more tender by a sort of "predigestion" which occurs.

It is postulated that nucleic acids are released when meat is ground, coming out with the meat juices, apparently making spoilage very fast by this means. Similar action may occur when ground meat is introduced into the intestinal tract. There the temperature is ideal for rapid spoilage. *This is particularly applicable if there is insufficient hydrochloric acid in the stomach*, as HCl acts as an intestinal antiseptic in inhibiting fermentation and putrefaction which might otherwise occur. **Here again, a proper digestive aid containing hydrochloric acid**

sources may be used to a distinct advantage.

Note: Preserved meats, such as wieners and sausages, do not have as much tendency to putrefaction since they contain anti-putrefactive chemicals (usually nitrites and/or nitrates) which work both inside and outside the body to produce this effect. However, for the same reason, they are not desirable from a nutritional viewpoint. It has been determined that these substances inhibit enzymes in the body, produce liver and kidney disease, as well as being possibly carcinogenic.

Regarding the Use of Sugar and Protein and/or Fat Combinations One of the little known deleterious effects of refined sugar is its reaction in the gastrointestinal tract with protein and/or fat combinations. First of all, let us establish that concentrated carbohydrates (sugars) stay in the stomach for only a short period of time since very little digestion is necessary.

On the other hand, proteins remain in the stomach for extended periods of time (up to 5 hours) because much activity must take place before the proteins can be passed on to the small intestine for absorption. Some fats also are broken down in the stomach and the presence of fat in the stomach slows down the production of hydrochloric acid, which further delays the time of departure of stomach contents. When concentrated carbohydrates are mixed with protein or protein/fat combinations, the sugars tend to ferment in the stomach, producing gas. Adequate hydrochloric acid will prevent this to some extent, but the major cause of stomach gas is improper combining of food groups. Too many Americans are accustomed to finishing off a good meal with sweet desserts. For best nutrition, concentrated sweets should be eaten on an empty stomach - this includes fruits, fruit juices, etc. as well.

There are many sugar-protein combinations which may be easily avoided if one is on the alert; an outstanding example is eggs with orange juice. The fact that many foods contain a combination of protein and carbohydrates must be taken into consideration, such natural combinations rarely give much trouble as it is the concentration of carbohydrates which produces the deleterious effects, these being proportional to the quantity present.

Regarding the Use of Fiber Foods in the Diet As a natural laxative, without griping, diarrhea, or any of the other complaints we have about most other laxatives, dietary fiber has no equal. Although many are not aware, they suffer from extremely slow movement of the digestive tract. There are many consequences of such slow tract time:

1. Intestinal gas because of the fermentation of starch and sugars.

2. Diverticulosis due to the large amounts of fecal material pushing against the wall of the intestine, producing little sacs or pouches which then fill with waste material. This is ideal circumstances for more

putrefaction to occur, which then discharges noxious matter into the tract which may be absorbed into the blood stream.

3. Hemorrhoids and varicosities can be blamed, at least in part, to the pressure exerted by the large amounts of material collected in the intestinal tract on the pelvic veins, creating back pressure which balloons the veins in the hemorrhoidal plexus and in the legs.

It would be a very apathetic individual indeed, who would not see the advantages of consuming some form of dietary fiber each and every day in order to help prevent the above from becoming a reality in his or her life. The Creative Restoration Diet suggests that one-half cup of whole grain bran flakes be consumed every day. These are not the processed bran flake cereals found in the supermarket, but 100% bran flakes usually found in health food stores. They can be mixed with granola, yogurt, salads, casseroles, etc. Bran or dietary fiber should not be referred to as "roughage" but rather as "softage" because it becomes a very soft, water-filled bulk in the intestines. The use of bran remedies the lack of fiber in a diet made up primarily of proteins (which contain very little fiber) and comparatively few raw fruits and vegetables.

Regarding the Use of Common Salt in the Diet People who use as much salt as they like, may excrete nine times as much potassium, an essential mineral, as those on salt-restricted diets. Actually, Americans frequently consume 20 to 25 times as much salt as estimated sodium requirements recommended. If this is not counter-balanced with increased potassium intake, a borderline potassium deficiency state is easily brought about.

Salt substitutes, mostly made up of potassium chloride, are often too bitter for anyone to stick with their use. We are fortunate in having a new 40-60 mixture of sodium and potassium chlorides on the market. This satisfies flavor requirements and you need not worry about the loss of potassium from using sodium chloride alone. This formula is available in most supermarkets and health food stores carry an expanded version which contains calcium, magnesium and lysine in addition to the basic potassium and sodium.

OVERALL PICTURE OF THE CREATIVE RESTORATION DIET

In order to help you obtain a better idea of the recommended diet, examples of "Desirable and Undesirable" foods are listed. Of course, not all foods in each category can be shown, but a study of the examples given will suffice to show the type of food necessary for best results.

DESIRABLE FOODS

1. **All Garden Vegetables** (fresh, frozen, canned, in order of desirability)

Asparagus	*Squash*
Peas	*Sprouts*

Parsley	Tomato
Cauliflower	Yams
Broccoli	Lettuce
Potatoes	Garbonzas
Parsnips	Cabbage
Corn	Celery
Rutabaga	Chard
Carrots	String Beans

2. Meat Dishes (veal, beef, lamb, venison, elk, buffalo, fish)

Steaks	Chops
Roast	Stew
Broiled	

3. Fermented Foods

Buttermilk	Yogurt
Cottage Cheese	Sauerkraut

4. Fruits, Fruit Juices, Vegetable Juice

All are acceptable - just be careful as to the combinations of fruits and/or fruit juices with proteins.

5. Nuts and Seeds

They are preferable in the raw state or dry roasted with little salt. They belong to the protein-fat category of foods.

6. Dietary Fiber

Wheat Bran	Oat Bran
Oatmeal	Agar-Agar
Psyllium Husk Powder	Pectin
Raw Vegetables	Raw Fruit

UNDESIRABLE FOODS

1. Commercially Processed Flour Products

White Breads	Crackers
Macaroni	White Buns
Pie Crusts	Doughnuts
Biscuits	Cookies
Dumplings	Cakes
White Rolls	Spaghetti

2. Commercially Processed White Sugar Products

Candy	Soda Pop
Pie	Pudding

3. Ground or Processed Meat

Hamburger	Meat Loaf
Chili	Potted Meat
Wieners	Sausage
Lunch Meats	Hash

(The exception to ground meat is when you grind it fresh and immediately use it.)

4. Sugar - Protein Combination

Ice Cream   *Chocolate Milk*
Baked Beans   *Desserts with Meals*
Milk Shakes
Fruits or fruit juices with meat, eggs or cheese

EMBRACING WHOLISTIC HEALTH

by Kurt W. Donsbach, D.C., N.D., Ph. D.

CLARIFYING THE
BODY - MIND - SPIRIT
CONNECTION
in
CANCER - ARTHRITIS - CANDIDIASIS
HEART DISEASE - MULTIPLE SCLEROSIS

Explicit treatment protocols from the world
famous natural healing institutions -
Hospital Santa Monica, Hospital St.
Augustine and Institut Santa Monica

You can order this 300 page, profusely illustrated manual by checking with your local health food store or by calling 1-800-423-7662. Total cost - $14.95. Dr. Donsbach feels this is his best work yet. You should have this book on your shelf to help you answer health questions that may come up. It is the best review of the application and merits of wholistic health philosophy available today.